Book 1:

Top Essential Oil Recipes

BY LINDSEY P

&

Book 2:

The Beginners Guide to Making Your Own Essential Oils

BY LINDSEY P

Book 1:

Top Essential Oil Recipes

BY LINDSEY P

A Recipe Guide Of Natural, Non-Toxic Aromatherapy & Essential Oils for Healing Common Ailments, Beauty, Stress & Anxiety

Table of Contents

Introduction

I want to thank you and congratulate you for purchasing the book, *"Top Essential Oil Recipes: A Recipe Guide Of Natural, Non-Toxic Aromatherapy & Essential Oils for Healing common ailments, beauty, Stress & Anxiety."*

This book contains proven steps and strategies on how to use and combine essential oils to help alleviate anxiety issues and address health and beauty concerns. You will also be introduced to the basics of essential oils, how they are produced, and how they must be used.

Thanks again for purchasing this book, I hope you enjoy it!

Chapter 1: What Are Essential Oils?

Have you ever squeezed a ripe orange peel? Surely you have noticed the fragrant residue on your hand? That residue is one example of an essential oil. Essential oils are naturally fragrant, highly concentrated compounds that can be obtained from myriad flowers, bark, roots, leaves, stems, seeds, and other plant parts. Each type of essential oil has their own characteristic scent that a person can immediately identify with one whiff.

Essential oils are fat soluble but they are not "oily" at all. They do not contain any fatty acids or lipids that are present in animal and vegetable oils. They also evaporate into the air unlike other oils. Essential oils are pure and very clean in a sense. When touched, it is immediately absorbed by the skin. Essential oils vary in colors. Untainted oils are usually translucent but some oils can be amber to deep blue in color.

Healing Effects of Essential Oils

Even though you might have heard of them recently, essential oils have actually been used for thousands of years. The ancient people rely on essential oils to heal and purify the body of ailments and diseases. When science and technology had taken over, the usage of these oils had greatly diminished since individuals have come to rely on drugs. But because of the myriad side effects of drugs, people are now opting for natural remedies including the use of essential oils. Apart from it medicinal properties, these powerful oils are also used for their cosmetic properties and emotionally uplifting benefits.

How to Use Essential Oils

Essential oils are not supposed to be applied directly on the skin unless appropriately diluted. This is because the potency of these oils can cause an allergic reaction on people with very sensitive skin. Here are some of the most common ways to use essential oils:

- Humidifier The essential oil's scent always calms and rejuvenates the senses. Alleviate symptoms of breathing in very dry air by adding a few drops of your favorite oil to a room humidifier. Not only will you breathe in scented, moist air but your asthma, sinusitis, and other related ailments will be put to a stop.

- Inhalation – If you don't have a humidifier, you can add a few drops of the essential oil into a small bowl of hot water. Put a towel over your head and inhale the aromatic steam vapors. If you have some trouble sleeping, you can strategically place a drop or two of the oil on your pillow to help relax yourself. If you are out of the home frequently, invest in a blank personal inhaler. This will allow you carry essential oil blends to rejuvenate or calm you anytime, anywhere.

- Bath Soak – Soaking in warm bathwater mixed with a few drops of essential oil helps remove stress, body pains, and heal minor skin diseases.

- Compress – Add about 5 drops (or more if you prefer) of essential oil to a small bowl of hot water. Soak a washcloth and wring out any excess. Place the towel on the part of your body that needs relief.

- Massage oil – Mixing a few drops of essential oil to a tablespoon of sweet almond oil, coconut oil, or grapeseed oil makes a perfect massage oil to soothe any bodily aches and pains.

- Diffuse – Instead of using a chemical-based air freshener, use essential oils instead. Place your oil inside a diffuser to dispense them into the hair. Not only will your home smell nice but you'll be relaxed as well.

- Dryer Sheet – Stop buying scented dryer sheets and make your own. Just add a few drops of your favorite oil fragrance to a piece of clean cloth and put in the dryer together with your clothes.

Chapter 2: Essential Oil Basics

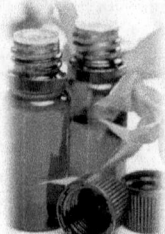

Now that you are showing an interest in essential oils, it is best that you, at least, know the basic things about them.

- It is very important to note that essential oils, although equally aromatic, are not the same with perfume and fragrance oils. Perfume and fragrance oils are created artificially, may contain chemicals, and don't have any therapeutic properties.

- Essential oils do not accumulate in the body. Once their healing properties are absorbed, they will be excreted naturally.

- Apart from water, essential oils can be diluted in carrier oils. Carrier oils are often unscented but others may have a faintly nutty or sweet fragrance. Perfect carrier oils for essential oils include sweet almond oil, pomegranate seed oil, evening primrose oil, olive oil, sesame oil, sunflower oil, hemp seed oil, jojoba, avocado oil, pecan oil, rose hip oil, and many more.

- Before using an essential oil for the first time, combine a drop of it to half a teaspoon of jojoba or olive oil. Rub the mixture on the inside of your wrist or upper arm. If there's no itching or redness after a few hours, the essential oil is safe for you to use. Remember, there's a great chance that you are allergic to essential oils if you have food allergies.

- Although most essential oils should never be used undiluted, small amounts of oils like lavender, tea tree, rose geranium, sandalwood, and German chamomile can be applied directly on the skin if used sparingly.

- Nursing women should steer clear from any type of essential oils. Pregnant women can use select oils sparingly only after the first trimester and upon the approval of a doctor.

- Never put essential oil on a baby or child's skin unless undiluted and half of the amount than a recipe calls for. Children have delicate, thin skin that may be damaged by the oil's potency. Essential oils that are safe for baby's include:

    a. Ginger

    b. Lemon

    c. Cypress

    d. Rosewood

      e. Rosemary

      f. Bergamot

      g. Roman Chamomile

      h. Lavender

      i. Orange

      j. Rose Otto

      k. Cedarwood

      l. Marjoram

      m. Mandarin

      n. Thyme

      o. Ylang-Ylang

      p. Melaleuca-Tea Tree

      q. Frankincense

      r. Geranium

      s. Sandalwood

- Essential oils can be tested of its purity. Pour a single drop on a piece of clean construction paper. It should evaporate quickly without any traces. If there's a noticeable ring, it means that the oil is diluted.

- Pure essential oils can last you 5 to 10 years depending on your usage. These oils are so potent that you'll only need a couple of drops for each use. Most oils stay potent even after a decade except for citrus oils, which may deteriorate after two years.

- Store all your essential oil in a dark glass container/bottle in a cool and dark place that's away from direct sunlight. This will help preserve their volume and potency.

- No matter how delicious these essential oils smell, you should never ingest it. These oils are meant to be used externally and not for consumption. If you have small children in the home, it is best to keep it away of their reach.

Chapter 3: Making Essential Oils

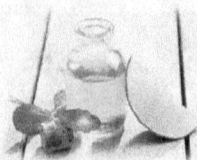

To make essential oils, it needs to be extracted from
the plant. This can be done through expression and
distillation.

Expression

Also referred as cold pressing, expression is method used to extract oils from
citrus fruits like lime, orange, tangerine, lemon, and bergamot. In the past,
expression doesn't require any sorts of tools except for a sponge. After soaking
the citrus rind or zest, it will be pressed against the sponge repeatedly to absorb
the oil. The sponge will then be squeezed over a container to catch the oils and
allow it to separate from its juices. After a few hours, the oils will be siphoned off
and bottled.

A modern type of expression involves using a blender-like device that's equipped
with spikes. Once the citrus zest, rind, or peel is placed into the device, it will
rotate and prod and prick the citrus until the oils are released. Oil will be
collected at the bottom of the device and bottled immediately.

Distillation

Most essential oils are extracted using the distillation process. In this process, the
plant part is placed on a grid that's inside a container called still. The still is then
sealed. The water, steam, or water/steam combination swirling inside the sealed
still will slowly break down the plant to release its volatile components and turn it
into steam. These components will then rise up and collect into the condenser.
Once the condenser is cool, the components will revert back into liquid form and
will be collected in a separate container. Once the essential oil separates from the
water, it will be siphoned off and stored.

Extraction

Essential oils can also be extracted by using alcohol. The dried plant material is
usually soaked in vodka or undenatured ethyl alcohol for several day until a
substantial amount of oil is produced.

DIY or Purchase?

When it comes to essential oils, is it advantageous to make your own or buy from
a trusted supplier?

Purchasing essential oils can get really expensive especially if you will be buying
several oils all at once. Although each bottle of essential oil will last a long time,
the amount that you pay upon the initial purchase can sting. The advantage of
buying essential oils from a reputable brand is that you can be sure of its potency
and quality.

Making your own essential oils is possible most especially if you have the time, patience, tools, and ingredients needed. If you already have everything you need, the cost of making your own essential oil will be minuscule. However, it is very important to note that DIY extraction of essential oils can lower its quality and potency unless you really are a pro. You would also need thousands of pounds of plant materials just to create a pound of a particular oil. You also need to make sure that it is very clean and free of chemicals like pesticides, herbicides, and the like.

All in all, it is best if you buy essential oils than make it yourself. Aside from being hassle-free, you can buy small quantities of several oils all at once. The more essential oils you have, the more chances you have of experiencing its benefits.'

Mixing and Matching Essential Oils

Now that you own several essential oils, you'll be glad to know that you can easily combine to create a concoction that can heal, relax, and beautify you. This powerful mixture is called a synergy blend. Synergy blend oils are combinations of different oils with complementing properties. These oil blends can be utilized for either aromatherapy, medicinal, or cosmetic purposes.

Chapter 4: Essential Oil Recipes for Various Ailments

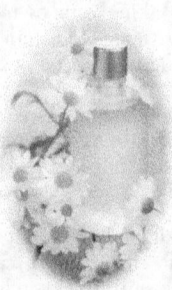

Pain

If you are in pain, concoct one of these essential oil recipes to get relief. Place all the needed oils in a small bottle, cap tightly, and shake well to mix. Then, massage on the affected areas (unless stated otherwise) whenever needed.

Nerve Pain

4 drops chamomile oil

3 drops helichrysum oil

3 drops marjoram oil

2 drops lavender oil

1 ounce St. John's wort oil

Stomach Pain

1 drop chamomile oil

1 drop peppermint oil

1 drop clove oil

2 drops rosemary oil

5ml vegetable carrier oil

Headaches

10 drops of peppermint oil

8 drops marjoram oil

10 drops basil oil

3 drops helichrysm oil

Injury

10 drops lavender oil

10 drops cypress oil

15 drops deep blue oil

10 drops sandalwood oil

20 drops marjoram oil

20 drops lemon grass oil

10ml vegetable carrier oil

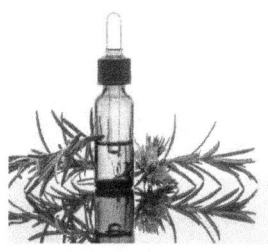

Pulled Muscle

2 drops sweet marjoram oil

3 drops Roman chamomile oil

*apply via cold compress

Muscle Pain

a. Blend 1

3 drops lavender oil

3 drops Roman chamomile oil

*apply via cold compress

b. Blend 2

5 drops rosemary oil

10 drops lavender oil

15 drops cypress oil

½ ounce sunflower oil

Tight Muscles

4 drops rosemary oil

4 drops lavender oil

2 drops ginger oil

4 teaspoons sweet almond oil

Sore Muscles

   a. **Blend 1**

5 drops peppermint oil

10 drops rosemary oil

5 drops Roman chamomile oil

5 drops lavender oil

5 drops lemon oil

1 ounce sweet almond oil

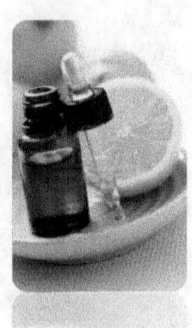

   b. **Blend 2**

20 drops Ylang-Ylang oil

12 drops nutmeg oil

20 drops ginger oil

8 drops rosemary oil

2   ounces sweet almond oil

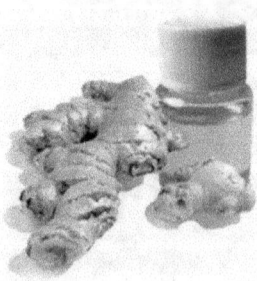

Blend 3

4 drops rosemary oil

4 drops bay laurel oil

3 drops Ylang-Ylang oil

4 drops eucalyptus oil

15ml carrier oil

Rheumatic Pain

4 drops ginger oil

2 drops spike lavender oil

4 drops silver fir oil

4 teaspoons carrier oil

Leg Cramps

2 drops ginger oil

4 drops cinnamon oil

4 drops black pepper oil

4 teaspoons carrier oil

Back Pains

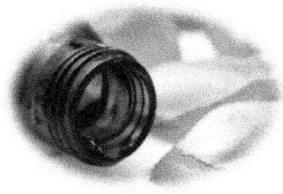

a. Blend 1

10 drops lavender oil

6 drops sandalwood oil

6 drops rosemary oil

3 drops geranium oil

2 tablespoons almond oil

b. Blend 2

4 drops cardamom oil

4 drops ginger oil

4 drops wintergreen

15ml sweet almond oil

For Assorted Health Concerns

Eczema Cream

25 drops Melrose oil

25 drops lavender oil

½ cup coconut oil (solid)

Put all the ingredients in a mixing bowl. Using a stand mixer, whip at medium-high speed until thick and peaky. Store the cream in small, wide-mouth glass jars. Apply on the skin before sleeping until skin condition improves.

Cough Blend

1 drop peppermint oil

1 drop pine needle oil

1 drop eucalyptus globulus

Put the oils in a small bowl of steaming hot water. Inhale the steam to loosen mucus and get relief.

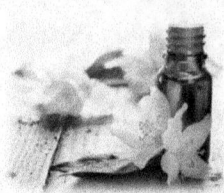

Cold Relief

2 drops rosemary oil

2 drops peppermint oil

2 drops eucalyptus globulus oil

Blend the oils together in a bottle and add a few drops in your personal inhaler. Place the inhaler near your nostrils and inhale slowly to get relief.

Fever Reducer

For kids 3 months to 6 years old:

5 drops chamomile oil

3 drops lavender oil

2 drops frankincense oil

For kids 6 to 10 years old:

2 drops frankincense

3 drops peppermint oil

5 drops rosemary oil

To use, place the selected oil blend in a steam vaporizer or oil diffuser. You can also dilute the oils with 1 ounce of carrier oil and apply it to the child's body.

Bruise Be Gone

8 drops helichrysum oil

1 ounce sweet almond oil

Put the oils in a bottle and shake well to combine. Apply lightly on the bruises several times a day.

Athlete's Foot Fighter

3 drops thyme oil

8 drops geranium oil

12 drops tea tree oil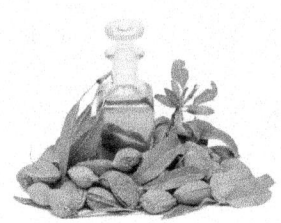

2 drops myrrh (optional)

2 ounces apple cider vinegar

1 tablespoon tincture of benzoin

Mix all the ingredients together and apply on the affected area. Apply several times a day.

Tooth Pain Relief

1 teaspoon vegetable oil

1 drop orange oil

4 drops clove bud oil

Combine the ingredients together. Rub on the gums every half hour or as needed. This recipe may also be used on children.

Sore Throat Gargle

½ cup warm water

4 drop marjoram oil

½ teaspoon sea salt

Combine all the ingredients in a cup. Stir well to dissolve the salt and break up oil. Gargle every 30 minutes each day to get relief.

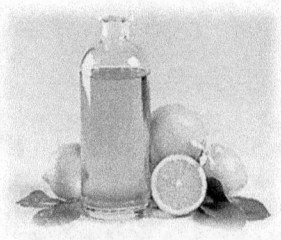

Herpes Relief

5 drops bergamot oil

5 drops myrrh oil

10 drops tea tree oil

2 drops peppermint oil (optional)

½ ounce vegetable oil

Combine all the ingredients and stir well. The addition of the peppermint oil in the recipe is optional as some people find that it increases the pain. If you can tolerate it, the better. Apply directly on the affected area several times a day.

Dermatitis Balm

8 drops chamomile oil

8 drops tea tree oil

2 ounces healing balm

1 teaspoon Oregon grape tincture

Use a toothpick to stir the oils and tincture into the healing balm. Once mixed, apply the balm 3 to 4 times a day to the afflicted area of the skin.

Inhalation Rub for Asthma

6 drops lavender oil

1 drop marjoram oil

4 drops geranium oil

1 drop ginger oil

1 ounce vegetable oil

Mix all the ingredients in a small bowl. Rub on the asthmatic's chest before bedtime and instruct him to inhale a few times before lying down. Repeat for several nights.

Bladder Infection Reliever

2 drops fennel oil

8 drops cypress oil

6 drops bergamot oil

6 drops tea tree oil

2 ounces vegetable oil

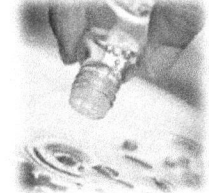

Mix all the ingredients and massage over your lower abdomen. You may also add a few drops of the oil blend to your warm bath.

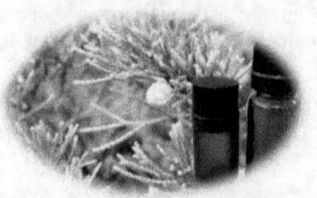

Chapter 5: Essential Oils Recipes for Stress and Anxiety

Mood Enhancer Natural Parfum

1 teaspoon fractionated coconut oil (melted)

1 drop bergamot oil

1 drop Ylang-Ylang oil

3 drops clary sage

4 drops tangerine oil

3 drops lavender oil

Put all the oils inside a roller bottle. Shake well before using.

Depression Lifter Spray

3 drops petitgrain Oil

6 drops bergamot oil

1 drop neroli oil (can be optional)

3 drops geranium oil

2 ounces water

Put all ingredients inside a spray bottle and shake well to blend. Spritz over your face or body whenever needed.

Anger Away Blend

4 drops Ylang-Ylang oil

3 drops cypress oil

2 drops frankincense oil

4 drops patchouli oil

2 drops clary sage

7 drops geranium

5 drops bergamot

Put all the ingredients inside a small bottle. Close and shake well. Rub small amounts of the oil over the heart and liver areas as well as on the bottoms of the feet.

For Emotional Release

15 drops sandalwood oil

25 drops geranium oil

30 drops Ylang-Ylang oil

10 drops ledum oil

20 drops German chamomile oil

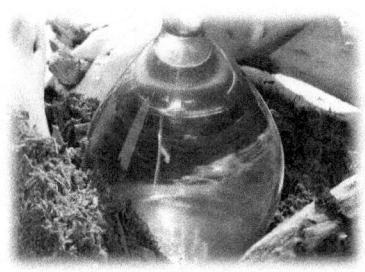

Put all the oils in a bottle. Secure cap and shake well. Rub a small amount on your chest and back.

Pick Me Upper

5 drops spearmint oil

10 drops bergamot oil

 10 drops grapefruit oil

Put all the oils in a bottle and mix well. Add several drops in a diffuser to lighten your mood.

Ease the Panic Blend

1 drop rose oil

20 drops bergamot oil

15 drops lavender oil

5 drops basil oil

3 drops neroli oil

Mix all the oils in a glass bottle by shaking vigorously. Put several drops in your personal inhaler whenever you feel panic settling in. You may also use a diffuser.

Slow Down Blend

1 drop lavender oil

1 drop Ylang-Ylang oil

1 drop bergamot oil

1 drop patchouli oil

Combine all the oils in a small bottle and shake well. Add a few drops in a diffuser to relax.

Comforting Body Spray

15 drops sweet orange oil

10 drops cinnamon leaf oil

8 ounces distilled water

1 tablespoon witch hazel

a spray bottle

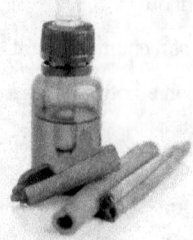

Pour all the ingredients inside the spray bottle. Close and shake well. Spray on your body whenever needed. Store in the fridge and use within two weeks.

Perk My Energy Blend

2 drops eucalyptus oil

2 drops peppermint oil

8 drops lemon oil

1 drop cinnamon leaf oil

1 drop cardamom oil

2 ounces vegetable oil

Combine all the ingredients and use to massage the entire body. Use as often as needed.

Memory Enhancer

1 drop clary sage oil

6 drops lemon oil

10 drops rosemary oil

Combine all the oils in a bottle and shake well. Add a few drops to your personal inhaler and smell while studying. You may also use the oil in your diffuser.

Sleep Inducer

10 drops sandalwood

10 drops lavender oil

15 drops bergamot oil

2 drops Ylang-Ylang oil

3 drops frankincense oil

4 ounces vegetable oil

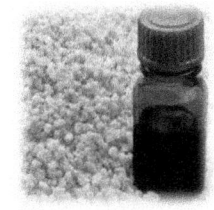

Mix all the ingredients together and massage all over the body. You can also add 2 teaspoons to your warm bath.

Chapter 6: Essential Oil Blends for Cosmetic Use

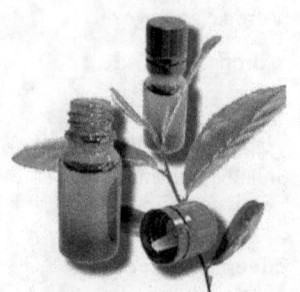

Make your own natural beauty products by using essential oils as ingredients. Try these recipes:

Peppermint Rosemary Shampoo

2 drops peppermint oil

16 drops rosemary oil

½ cup distilled water

½ cup castile soap

Obtain a clean flip top container and put in the castile soap. Add the peppermint and rosemary oil before adding the water. Close the container and shake before using.

Oily Skin Toner

1 drop rose geranium oil

3 drops palmarosa oil

3 drops lemongrass oil

3 drops petitgrain oil

3 drops tea tree oil

1 cup witch hazel

Mix all the ingredients and apply on the face using a cotton ball. Let dry.

Honey Lavender Lip Balm

15 drops lavender oil

5 drops Frankincense oil

1 tablespoon sweet almond oil

½ teaspoon raw honey

2 tablespoon coconut oil

2 tablespoon beeswax

1 tablespoon raw honey

1 rubber band (large)

12 lip balm tubes

Remove the caps from all tubes and position them upright using the rubber band. Using a double broiler, melt the honey, coconut oil, shea butter, and beeswax. Remove from heat once melted and mix in the essential oils and sweet almond oil. Carefully pour the mixture into the tubes, dividing them equally. Let the balm set before recapping the tubes.

Extra Strength Blemish Mask

800 units Vitamin E

12 drops tea tree oil

½ teaspoon Oregon grape root powder

Several drops of water

Stir the oil into the powder. Add water by drop until a paste is formed. Apply the mask on the entire face and let dry. Wait for 20 minutes before rinsing.

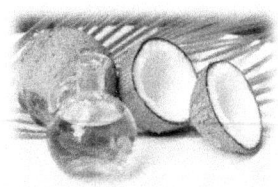

Shaving Cream

12 drops pure lavender oil

2 tablespoons sweet almond oil

3 tablespoons coconut oil

4 tablespoon shea butter (solid)

Use a double broiler to melt the coconut oil and shea butter over a low heat. Stir until completely melted. Add the remaining oils and mix well. Put in the fridge and let harden for a few hours. Remove from the fridge and whip until a frosting-like consistency is achieved. Let it sit for a few minutes before transferring to an airtight jar.

Lemon Honey Body Scrub

¼ cup olive oil

15 drops lavender oil

15 drops lemon oil

2 teaspoons dried rosemary

2 tablespoons raw honey

1 cup organic cane sugar

Mix the rosemary, raw honey, and sugar with the olive oil. Add in the essential oils and stir thoroughly. Use immediately or you can store it in a glass container for later use. This scrub lasts up to 2 to 3 months.

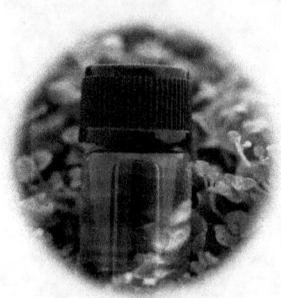

Homemade EO Toothpaste

20 drops peppermint oil

10 drops trace minerals

2 tablespoons coconut oil

2 tablespoons calcium magnesium powder

2 tablespoons baking soda

2 tablespoons real sea salt

2 tablespoons xylitol powder

Mix all powdered ingredients first. Add the coconut oil one tablespoon at a time. Add the salt and the peppermint oil. Mix thoroughly and store in a jar with a secure lid.

Solid Perfumes

- **Deep and Sensual Scent**

    10 drops sandalwood oil

    20 drops sweet orange oil

    15 drops Ylang-Ylang oil

- **Fresh and Spicy Scent**

    10 drops vetiver oil

17 drops grapefruit oil

14 drops ginger oil

- **Romantic and Whimsical Scent**

10 drops vetiver oil

25 drops rose oil

10 drops lime oil

Choose the scent of your choice and prepare the essential oils needed. Use double broiler and melt 2 teaspoon grated beeswax. Turn off the heat and add in 2 teaspoon sweet almond oil. Mix well and add the appropriate essential oils. Pour the mixture into your desired container and let harden. To use: rub a finger into the solid perfume before wiping it on your skin.

Soothing Natural Deodorant

3 tablespoons apricot kernel oil

5 tablespoons coconut oil

2 tablespoons dried calendula

3 tablespoons dried chamomile

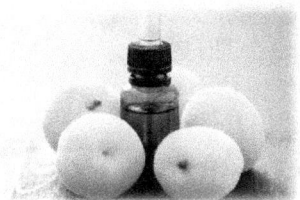

10 drops tea tree oil

10 drops lavender oil

¼ cup + 2 tablespoons arrow root powder

¼ cup + 2 tablespoons baking soda

Liquefy the coconut oil using a double broiler or the microwave. Put it in a sterilized jar and add in the apricot kernel oil. Put in the dried calendula and dried chamomile in the jar and seal tightly. Shake well until the flowers are completely soaked. Store in a dark place for 3 weeks, shaking the jar daily.

After the appropriate time, strain the infused oil and remove the flowers. You may need to heat up the oil if it has solidified. In another jar, mix the infused oil, the arrow root powder, and baking soda. Mix well. Add the essential oils per drop while stirring. Use within 3 months.

Hair Styling Wax

10 drops rosemary oil

10 drops peppermint oil

0.75 ounce beeswax

0.75 ounce fractionated coconut oil

0.5 ounce shea butter

Put the beeswax, coconut oil, and shea butter in a double broiler. Stir until completely melted. Turn off the heat and let cool for about 3 minutes. Add the oils and mix well. Transfer the mixture into a lidded glass jar. Let rest for two hours before using. Using your fingers, apply a small amount on the hair and style as usual.

Natural Sunscreen

1 teaspoon vitamin E

2 tablespoons zinc oxide

12 drops helichrysum oil

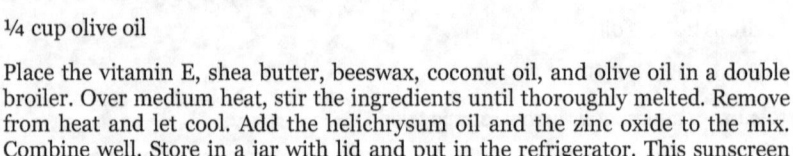

2 tablespoons shea butter

¼ cup beeswax

¼ cup fractionated coconut oil

¼ cup olive oil

Place the vitamin E, shea butter, beeswax, coconut oil, and olive oil in a double broiler. Over medium heat, stir the ingredients until thoroughly melted. Remove from heat and let cool. Add the helichrysum oil and the zinc oxide to the mix. Combine well. Store in a jar with lid and put in the refrigerator. This sunscreen must be used within 6 months of creation.

Talc-Free Powder

½ cup arrowroot powder

½ cup cornstarch

½ cup oats (finely ground)

2 drops lavender oil

1 drop Roman chamomile oil

Mix all the ingredients well and store in a shaker bottle.

Moisturizing Facial Oil

Base oils:

Argan oil (for aging, dry, oily, and acne-prone skin)

Jojoba oil (for aging, dry, oily, and acne-prone skin)

Grapeseed oil (for normal, oil, and acne-prone skin)

Nourishing oils:

Sea buckthorn oil – nourishing and perfect for all skin types

Rosehip seed oil – regenerating, firming, and perfect for all skin types especially aging skin

Borage oil – perfect for oily and acne-prone skin

Evening primrose skin – perfect for all skin types

Essential Oils:

Lavender – a healing oil that's perfect for all skin types

Peppermint – astringent oil that's perfect for oily and acne-prone skin

Rose – components are suitable for dry, aging, and normal skin.

Rosemary – for acne-prone and oily skin

Choose one of each base oil, nourishing oil, and essential oil that's suitable for your skin type. Fill a 1-ounce bottle and fill the bottle almost halfway with your base oil. Add in your nourishing oil. The bottle should be almost full at this time. Lastly, add 5 to 7 drops of the essential oil of your choice. If using peppermint, you might want to add only about 3 to 4 drops. Shake well. Store away from direct sunlight and use within one year.

Dry Shampoo

2 drops peppermint oil

2 drops rosemary oil

2 drops lavender oil

*¼ cup arrowroot powder

*for dark hair, use 2 tablespoons arrowroot powder and 2 tablespoons of cocoa powder

Combine all ingredients in a food processor. Pulse until thoroughly blended. Store in a wide mouth jar. Apply the powder to the roots of the hair using an old makeup brush.

Nail and Cuticle Care

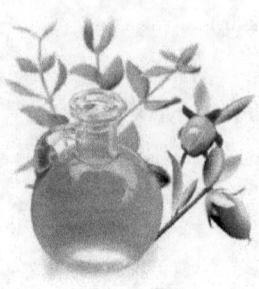

3 drops lemon oil

3 drops geranium oil

3 drops rosemary oil

6 drops clary sage

6 drops lavender

1 ounce sweet almond oil

1 ounce jojoba

Put all the oil inside a bottle and shake to blend well. At bedtime, put a drop on each of your fingernail and massage. This will help soften the cuticles and harden the nails.

Anti-Itch Lotion

10 drops German chamomile

20 drops lavender

5 drops peppermint

10 eucalyptus globulus

Mix all the oils together and add to **2 ounces of lotion** (unscented). Stir well. Apply to itchy area to get relief.

Conclusion

Thank you again for purchasing this book!

I hope this book was able to help you to understand essential oils and their many uses.

The next step is to continue experimenting with different essential oil blends and find your signature scent and cure.

Finally, if you enjoyed this book, please take the time to share your thoughts and post a review on Amazon. We do our best to reach out to readers and provide the best value we can. Your positive review will help us achieve that. It'd be greatly appreciated!

Thank you and good luck!

Book 2:

The Beginners Guide to Making Your Own Essential Oils

BY LINDSEY P

Complete Guide to Making Your Own Essential Oils from Scratch & To Improve Your Health and Well-Being

Table of Contents

Introduction

I want to thank you and congratulate you for purchasing the book, *The Beginners Guide To Making Your Own Essential Oils: Complete Guide To Making Your Own Essential Oils From Scratch & To Improve Your Health And Well-Being.*

This book contains proven steps and strategies on how to make your very own essentials oils to keep you healthy and away from many diseases and sicknesses.

Since the beginning of time, aromatherapy has been used by our ancestors to promote health, for medical practice and for personal hygiene. Aromatherapy uses essential oils extracted from flowers, stems, leaves, barks and other parts of a plant. These essential oils are believed to enhance physical as well as psychological well-being.

The aroma of these essential oils is believed to stimulate brain function when inhaled. Essential oils are also absorbed through the skin easily, wherein they promote well-being and healing by travelling through the bloodstream.

More and more people are discovering the medicinal benefits of aromatherapy, which is why it is gaining popularity really fast. Aromatherapy is used in various applications including increased cognitive function, enhanced mood and pain relief.

There are numerous essential oils and aromatherapy products available. Each of them has their own healing properties.

This book explains what essential oils are and how they are made. Inside, you will also discover various essential oils and the benefits that they offer. You can use this book as a guide on how to use aromatherapy and which essential oil is best to use for a specific condition.

Thanks again for purchasing this book, I hope you enjoy it!

Chapter 1

What Are Essential Oils

Essential oils are extracted from leaves, flowers, barks, stems, roots and other parts of a plant, commonly by steam. Essential oils are commonly clear but may also have amber, yellow or deep blue color. Essential oils are also referred to as essences since they contain the true essence of the plant where they are extracted from. Although essential oils have pleasing aromatic scents, they are different from fragrance oils.

Unlike fragrance oils, essential oils are pure and do not contain artificial fragrances or substances, that is why fragrance oils are not suitable for aromatherapy. Essential oils are used for its therapeutic benefits since the beginning of recorded history. These essential oils are usually inhaled or applied to the skin for absorption. History has proven the psychological and physical therapeutic benefits of essentials oils, although no scientific evidence has proven it.

Since essential oils are either inhaled or applied directly to the skin, you should take time to check if you have any allergic reactions to any of them. Apply a small amount to the side of your hand and wait for a few hours for any allergic reactions. Moreover, if you are allergic to the source plant, fruit or seed, chances are, you are also allergic to the essential oil extracted from it.

Although they are called "essential oils", they are not really oils. Unlike actual oil, essential oils do not contain fatty acids which make them actual oil. Furthermore, essential oils are volatile and they evaporate when left uncovered. Essential oils are often diluted in carrier oils such as grape seed oil, sweet almond oil and apricot kernel oil. You can buy essential oils individually bottled in small bottles. Most essential oils are sold as blends of various essential oils such as the Thieves essential oil. This essential oil is a combination of clove, lemon, cinnamon, eucalyptus and rosemary essential oils.

Chapter 2

An Easy Way to Make Your Own Essential Oil At Home

Essential oils are generally extracted from plants through distillation, commonly using steam. But other processes are also used such as solvent extraction, florasols extraction and expression. Essential oils are greatly used in perfumes, soaps and cosmetics. They are also used to flavor food and drinks and to add scent to household cleaning products and incense.

One of the most popular and easiest essential oil to make at home is the orange essential oil. Orange peels usually end up in the garbage and are just wasted. Instead of buying expensive scents, you can make your very own citrus scent at home without spending too much. Furthermore, making your own essential oil means you are guaranteed to be using a 100% natural product, free from harmful chemicals.

This procedure is an example of extracting essential oil using alcohol.

All you need are the following:

Orange peels (remove most of the white pith as possible)

Glass jar or glass bottle with a tight lid

Vodka (No need for the expensive ones. Any cheap vodka will do)

Undenatured Ethyl alcohol (as a substitute for the Vodka)

Coffee filter (cheesecloth or muslin will do)

Paper towel (muslin or cheesecloth can also be used as a substitute)

Dry your orange peels in a warm, dry place but away from direct sunlight until they are hard and dry. It usually takes 2 days for this but you can cut the orange peels into smaller pieces to help dry them faster.

Place the dried orange peels into the glass jar or bottle. Place the bottle of vodka or undenatured ethyl alcohol into a bowl of hot tap water for a few minutes then pour it into the jar/bottle of dried orange peels until they are all soaked. Cover the jar/bottle tightly and shake it vigorously for 2 to 3 minutes. Do this three to four times a day for 3 days or more. The more you shake the mixture and the longer you leave the orange peels soaked, the more oil you can extract.

Using a coffee filter or cheesecloth, strain the orange peels into a bowl. Cover it with cheesecloth or paper towel. Do not let the towel/cloth fall into the liquid as it will seep it and you will lose your essential oil.

Let the liquid sit for a few days in a cool, dark and clean area until all the alcohol has evaporated. Now you have pure orange essential oil that you can use for fragrance, soaps, candles, lotion, potpourris or aromatic waters.

When extracting essential oil from leaves or flowers using undenatured ethyl alcohol or vodka, the process is almost the same as above. The only difference is, when you strain the flowers/leaves from the mixture, you need to gently press them to release more oil. Furthermore, while you are soaking them in alcohol or vodka, you can add more leaves or flowers until you are able to reach your desired strength for your essential oil.

Chapter 3

How to Make Your Own Essential Oil At Home through Distillation

The most popular way of extracting essential oil from plants is through distillation. Normally, you need an apparatus called the still to be able to collect essential oil from plants. But, if you do not have distillation equipment and you want to create your own essential, it is still possible. The yield may not be as great as when you are using a still and the process may be longer but it's a great alternative.

You will need a crock pot, some distilled water, air-tight glass container, bowl and cheesecloth. This procedure is very simple but it takes time.

- Decide what plant material you want to extract essential oil from. Dry your plant material. Make sure not to over dry them and do not place them under direct sunlight as it may lose some of its essential oils.

- Place your dried plant material into the crock pot and fill it with distilled water until all the plant material is soaked.

- Cook in low heat for 24 hours. Do not attempt to increase the heat to make the process faster as it will affect the quality and yield of the essential oil.

- Leave crock pot open until cool. Cover with cloth and let it sit in a cool, dry place for a week. You will see oil separating on top of the water in the crock pot. Collect the oil off and place it in a dark, tightly covered container.

- Cover the container with cheesecloth and allow the rest of the water to evaporate. This will take about a week.

- You now have your very own essential oil made possible through distillation at home.

Another distillation method that can be done at home is by grounding up your dried plant material. Use a cotton or linen bag as a container for your ground plant material for cooking. Make sure to tie the bag shut so that no plant material falls off during the process.

Put some distilled water in a crock pot, enough to soak up the bag of plant material. Bring it to a boil. When the water is already boiling, reduce the heat to low and let it simmer for 24 hours.

Let the water cool. You will notice some oil on the surface of the water. Collect the oil and place in a clean, dry, dark glass container. Squeeze the bag unto the water in the crock pot and collect the oil from the surface.

Cover the glass container with clean cloth (cheesecloth or cotton preferably). Let it sit in a cool, dry place for a week to allow the excess water to evaporate.

You can now enjoy your very own essential oil.

Chapter 4

How to Use Oil to Extract Essential Oil

Extracting essential oil using is very and can be done from home. It is most ideal to use almond oil, Jojoba oil or grapeseed for this process. Do not use a metal container when using oils to extract essential oils from plant materials as it will affect the quality of the essential oil. Use non-metallic containers only such as ceramic crock or glass containers.

This process is best used for herbs and flowers such as rosemary, lavender, rose or the likes. You may or may not dry your herb or flowers. It all depends on you. Drying can reduce the amount of essential oil from your herb/flower but it can help increase your yield per batch as you will be able to cramp in more herbs/flowers per batch.

Things you will need:

Large glass bottle

Extracting oil (grapeseed, almond or jojoba)

Cheesecloth

Procedure:

Fill half of the large glass bottle with your extracting oil (carrier oil) such as jojoba, rapeseed or almond). Put as much herbs/flowers/leaves into the glass bottle. Make sure that all the plant materials are completely submerged into the oil. Cover the glass tightly with its lid and let sit for 24 hours in a cool, dark, clean area.

Shake the mixture from time to time within three days. You can do this three to four times each day. Shaking will help extract more oil from the plant material.

After three days, strain the plant material. Use a ceramic bowl to catch the oil from the glass bottle. You can add more plant materials into the oil if the scent is not strong enough for you. Remember, you have to let it sit for 24 hours and repeat all the process after that.

Place your extracted essential oil in a dark, clean container. This essential oil is ready to use.

Another way of extracting essential oil from a plant material using oil is by slow cooking. Here's how to do it:

- In a crock pot, place 2 cups of olive oil (jojoba, rapeseed or almond) and mix ½ ounce of plant material (flowers, leaves, herbs, etc) into it.

- Slow cook the mixture in low heat for up to 6 hours. You may stir the mixture a few times to ensure that the plant materials are completely soaked into the carrier oil (olive oil, jojoba, rapeseed, almond).

- Leave the crock pot open to cool the mixture.

- Strain the oil mixture using an unbleached cheese cloth. Use a ceramic bowl to place the oil while straining.

- Place the essential oil in a dark, clean, tightly covered glass bottle and use sparingly.

Another easy way of extracting essential oil from plant materials using is by grounding the plant materials and soaking them in carrier oils. This process takes a long time of waiting but it's fairly easy to do.

First, dry your plant material. Do not expose your plant material in direct sunlight as it will lose most of its essential oils. Dry in a dark, cool place for about 2 days. Do not over dry. When the plant material is already wilted and dried, it's ready to be grounded.

After grinding the plant material, take one tablespoon and place it in a clear, glass bottle or jar. Add ½ cup of carrier oil (olive oil, rapeseed, almond, jojoba) and ½ teaspoon white vinegar. Stir to combine all the ingredients. Cover the glass bottle/jar and leave it in a warm, sunny area for three weeks. Make sure to place the bottle in an area where there is plenty sunlight. Shake the bottle two to three times a day for three weeks.

Strain the mixture and place your essential oil in a dark, glass container. Please note that essential oils are very pure so they must be used in small amounts only.

To ensure that you are not allergic to any essential oils, perform the skin patch test. Place a small amount of essential oil on the side of your palm. Wait for a few hours. If no irritation, itchiness or swelling occurs, you are not allergic to the essential oil and you may continue using it. In general, if you are allergic to the herb, flower or fruit of a certain plant, you are most likely allergic to its essential oil as well.

Chapter 5

Essential Oils: Uses and Benefits

The use of essential oils and making your own at home can be very fun, fulfilling and beneficial therapeutically. Always remember that essential oils are not meant to be swallowed or ingested. There may be some essential oils that are safe to ingest, but even so, you still need to consult an expert before ingesting any essential oils.

Essential oils are commonly inhaled. For first timers, you can place one to two drops of your desired essential oil in a piece of tissue and carefully inhale the scent. Those who are already veterans in using essential oils usually place a small amount of essential oil on their palm and rub it a little, and then they cover their nose with their palm and inhale the aroma of the essential oil.

When you are suffering from colds or influenza, the best way to treat your condition with essential oils is through steam inhalation. Pour 2 cups of boiled water in a bowl and add 3 to 7 drops of essential oil into it. You may lessen the number of drops if you are using essential oils with strong scents that may irritate your mucus membranes. Some of these essential oils include thyme, rosemary, cinnamon, pine eucalyptus, cajuput and others. Do not place your nose too near the bowl. Put at least about 10 to 12 inches gap between the bowl and your nose. Inhale the steam gradually and carefully. Do not inhale constantly as it may irritate your nose. If you feel any discomfort or irritation, discontinue use right away. This can be done anytime, day or night.

Please note that too much inhalation of essential oils can cause dizziness, vertigo, lethargy, nausea and headaches. Although essential oils are greatly used to treat respiratory problems and sinuses, you must take precaution when using them. Do not use over 10 drops. Aside from hot water, you may also use diffusers or hot compress for inhalation.

Essential oils are also great for making your room smell fresh. To expel any unwanted smell in your house, you may sprinkle a few drops of essential oils in your trash can, drain, vacuum bag filter or laundry wash. You may also add a few drops on your tissue before you keep them in your cabinet. Please take note that essential oils are flammable. Do not place them near fire or too much heat.

Essential oils are also great insect repellents. Essential oils of citronella, peppermint and lavender are natural insect repellents. To prevent insects from infesting your household, place a few drops on a cotton ball and place it on your doorway, windows and other areas where you frequently see insects. If you are a pet owner, some essential oils are not suitable for pets. Some of these essential oils include anise, garlic, juniper, horseradish, clove leaf or clove bud, thyme, Wintergreen, yarrow and others.

On the contrary, there are also some essential oils that are used for pets, especially for dogs due to their calming effects. Most common of these are chamomile, eucalyptus, lavender, ginger, myrrh, rose, valerian, cedarwood atlas, ravensare and others. Essential oils are usually used for pet baths and for calming the pet's nerves through diffusion.

Remember that your pet cannot tell you if it is or is not working. Always check for signs of irritation as excessive scratching, too much whining, sniffing and nervousness. If any of these signs are present, discontinue use.

Either for humans or for pets always dilute your essential oil. For pets, essential oils are best diluted at 25% of human formula. Never use essential oils internally for your pets. Size matters for essential oils. Smaller pets should be given smaller amount of essential oil. But even if your pet is huge, let's say a horse; less is still better with essential oils. Birds and fish should never be given essential oils. Birds are highly sensitive and cannot tolerate essential oils just as fish cannot tolerate floral waters or oils.

Essential oils are also greatly used for a relaxing massage. Do not use any essential oil that is not diluted as it may cause skin irritations. Use 1 ounce of carrier oil such as almond oil and add 10 to 20 drops of essential oil. Do not apply on the genitals and near the eyes.

Essential oils are also popularly used for soaps, shampoos, lotions, shower gels, facial toners and perfumes for their great aroma and therapeutic benefits.

If you are experiencing circulatory problems, skin problems, respiratory symptoms, menstrual pain, muscle pain or stress and nervous tension, an aromatic bath will give you great relief. Please be aware that essential oils should be mixed with either salt or emulsifier like sesame oil or milk before they can be safely dispersed into the water. Essential oils will float on water if not mixed with salt or emulsifier and will directly get into the skin which can cause irritations.

Aromatic bath uses warm water and essential oils that are not mixed with salt or emulsifier can cause dermotoxicity especially if the essential oil used is of a heating nature. For safety purposes, avoid spicy oils in your bath. These essential oils include thyme, tulsi, oregano and cinnamon oil. Also, avoid phototoxic oils such as bergamot oil and citrus oils. Essential oils with specific irritant potential such as lemongrass should also be avoided. Essential oils that are generally considered mild for use in baths are:

- Lavender oil

- Clary Sage oil

- Rose oil

- Geranium oil

- Frankincense oil

44

- Sandalwood oil

- Eucalyptus oil

- Cedar oil

- Fir oil

- Pine oil

- Pinon pine essential oil

- Spruce oil

- Juniper oil

Combine 5 to 10 drops of essential oil in ½ to 1 cup of salt or emulsifier and add it into your warm bath. Do not soak too long in aromatic water. The ideal soaking time is between 10 to 15 minutes only. Soaking too long under aromatic baths may cause skin irritation and other symptoms such as headache and nausea.

If you suffer from dysmenorrhea or menstrual cramps, skin problems and muscle aches or if you have a wound or a bruise, you can use essential oil (lavender, thieves, Melrose) compress for relief. Just add 10 drops of essential oil in 4oz of warm water and soak a clean cloth in it. Wring the cloth gently and place it on the affected area. Repeat the process for 10 to 15 minutes.

For relief from inflammation, you may use the following essential oils for your compress:

- Wintergreen – This essential oil has a warming effect. Its methyl salicylate and cortisone-like effect reduces inflammation and pain in the muscles and joints.

- Helichrysum – This essential oil has powerful anti-inflammatory properties making it ideal for cuts and bruises. It also helps boost circulation and cleanses the blood.

- Clove – This essential oil helps relieve pain due to arthritis and rheumatism. It has anti-infectious properties as well as anti-inflammatory, anesthetic and antiseptic properties which also make it ideal for wounds, scrapes and bruises.

- Peppermint – For pain, peppermint essential oil is great. It has pain blocking properties, antispasmodic and anti-inflammatory properties. It provides cooling and soothing effects and it also dilates the respiratory system.

- Palo Santo – Due to its anticoagulant and anti-inflammatory properties, this essential oil is excellent for relieving tired muscles and joints. It is also rich in limonene, an antioxidant.

- Lemon – Essential oil extracted from lemon has antiseptic properties which make it great for wounds and cuts. It also has immune-stimulating properties which uplifts your mood.

- Copal/Copaiba – This essential oil has excellent anti-inflammatory properties which are good for wounds, cuts and bruises. It is also an antiseptic, antibacterial and analgesic. Furthermore, Copaiba/Copal essential oil helps boost the respiratory, nervous and cardiovascular systems.

Essential oils are also used for massage due to their calming and warming effects as well as their therapeutic benefits. Take note that essential oils are pure and must be diluted in carrier oils before use. For adults, it is ideal to place 12 drops of essential oil in an ounce of carrier oil. For children under 12 years old, it is generally safe to use 6 drops of essential oil in an ounce of carrier oil. You may lessen the number of drops for the essential oils especially if you are just starting.

Chapter 6

List of Essential Oils and Their Uses

There are so many essential oils out in the market and there are even more that are yet to be discovered. Below is a quick guide to essential oils and their uses.

- Basil – This essential oil is antiviral, antibacterial, antispasmodic and anti-inflammatory. It is also a muscle relaxant, stimulant, decongestant and antiseptic. Due to its therapeutic properties, basil essential oil is often used to treat migraines, muscle aches and pains, mental fatigue, anxiety, depression, throat and lung infections, bronchitis, menstrual cramps, dandruff and insect bites. It can also be used as an insect repellant for flies and mosquitoes.

  You may dilute it in carrier oil such as vegetable or coconut oil. A 50:50 dilution is ideal, meaning one part basil essential oil is to one part carrier oil. You may apply the diluted basil essential oil in the problem areas or inhale it by placing 1 to 2 drops on the palm of your hand rubbing it lightly. If you are asthmatic, do not inhale any essential oil. Instead, place it on the sole of your feet. You may also diffuse it by using the candle method or the steam method.

- Bergamot – Bergamot is known for its relaxing and uplifting effect and has a sweet and fruity scent. It is used to help fight addiction and to relieve stress, anxiety and depression. It is also know to relieve infections such as herpes and vaginal candida as well as cold sores, urinary tract infections and respiratory infections. You may use diluted Bergamot essential oil for massage or apply topically on the affected area. You can also diffuse it or inhale it by adding a few drops on your palm.

- Clary Sage – The sharp, grassy and spicy aroma of Clary Sage essential oil helps relax the mind. It helps prevent hair loss by boosting hair growth. It is an antioxidant, astringent and antiseptic making it effective in preventing wrinkles and keeps skin healthy (for dry and oily skin). It helps relieve menstrual problems and PMS, pre-menopausal symptoms, insomnia, impotence, hemorrhoids, bronchitis, high cholesterol and kidney disorders.

- Chamomile – Chamomile essential oil can tone the skin through continued use. It is also a known anti-depressant and reduces nervousness.

- Cinnamon – For the relief of joint pains and improved circulation, cinnamon essential oil is greatly advised. It also helps reduce nervousness by calming the nerves.

- Cucumber – Essential oil extracted from cucumber is an excellent detoxifier and skin moisturizer. It also helps reduce puffiness of the eyes. The calming effect of cucumber essential oil is great for relaxing the mind and body.

- Eucalyptus – This essential oil is effective in killing lice. Dilute one part eucalyptus essential oil to one part coconut oil and apply to hair. Leave for 5 to 10 minutes only. Rinse off with water or shampoo. It also eases joint and muscle pains and clears respiratory passages.

- Jasmine – This is a must-have for girls. Jasmine essential oil reduces scars and helps relieve PMS symptoms. It is also effective in relieving muscle spasms and for treating dry and sensitive skin.

- Lavender – This essential oil is best known for its calming effect making it an effective treatment for insomnia and stress. It also reduces symptoms of PMS.

- Lemon – Lemon essential oil is known to clear respiratory passages making it effective for the treatment of colds and other respiratory problems. The antibacterial and antiseptic properties of lemon essential oil also make it an effective treatment for acne. It also boosts the immune system, treat dandruff and helps lower down fever.

- Orange – Essential oil from orange has anti-inflammatory properties which relieve pain and inflammation. It is also an anti-depressant and an aphrodisiac.

- Peppermint – For fast relief of headache, peppermint essential oil is highly recommended. It also relieves nausea and decreases indigestion. It also eases clogged nose and relieves other respiratory problems.

- Sage – Sage essential oil heals wounds, fights infections and calms upset stomach.

Always remember to store your essential oils in a cool dry place and away from direct sunlight and heat as it may lose its potency and its quality can be compromised.

Conclusion

Thank you again for purchasing this book!

I hope this book was able to help you learn how to make your own essential oil from scratch and know more about the uses and benefits of essential oils.

The next step is to start making your own essential oils and start living a healthier and stress-free life.

Finally, if you enjoyed this book, please take the time to share your thoughts and post a review on Amazon. We do our best to reach out to readers and provide the best value we can. Your positive review will help us achieve that. It'd be greatly appreciated!

Thank you and good luck!

Check Out My Other Books

Below you'll find some of my other popular books that are popular on Amazon and Kindle as well.   Simply click on the links below to check them out. Alternatively, you can visit my author page on Amazon to see other work done by me.

Coconut Oil for Easy Weight Loss

http://amzn.to/1i5f45p

Essential Oils & Aromatherapy

http://amzn.to/1ouuZTx

Superfoods that Kickstart Your Weight Loss

http://amzn.to/1eyHdku

The Best Secrets Of Natural Remedies

http://amzn.to/1gmHd7y

The Hypothyroidism Handbook

http://amzn.to/1emWfyR

The Hyperthyroidism Handbook

http://amzn.to/1kqLQCp

Essential Oils & Weight Loss For Beginners

http://amzn.to/Q83bFp

Top Essential Oil Recipes

http://amzn.to/1lSrhSC

Soap Making For Beginners

http://amzn.to/1fkmYwr

Body Butters For Beginners

http://amzn.to/1fWjwJe

Homemade Body Scrubs & Masks For Beginners

http://amzn.to/1jjLRIO

Carrier Oils For Beginners

http://amzn.to/1sbqUQP

Natural Homemade Cleaning Recipes For Beginners

http://amzn.to/1izDB2m

The Beginners Guide To Medicinal Plants

http://amzn.to/1vSujr6

The Beginners Guide To Making Your Own Essential Oils

http://amzn.to/1piUNSB

The Beginners Alkaline Miracle Diet

http://amzn.to/1sDVaVE

Thyroid Diet

http://amzn.to/1piW2RY

Essential Oils Box Set #1 (Weight Loss + Essential Oil Recipes

http://amzn.to/1qlYWWP

Essential Oils Box Set #2 (Weight Loss + Essential Oil & Aromatherapy

http://amzn.to/1qlYWWP

Essential Oils Box Set #3 Coconut Oil + Apple Cider Vinegar

http://amzn.to/1oIFZJw

Essential Oils Box Set #4 Body Butters & Top Essential Oil Recipes

http://amzn.to/1jSxURJ

Essential Oils Box Set #5 Soap Making & Homemade Body Scrubs

http://amzn.to/RAvJYo

Essential Oils Box Set #6 Body Butters & Body Scrubs

http://amzn.to/RAvSel

Essential Oils Box Set #7 Top Essential Oils & Best Kept Secrets Of Natural
Remedies

http://amzn.to/1gvsRCq

Essential Oils Box Set #8 Homemade Cleaning Recipes & Essential Oil Recipes

http://amzn.to/1gxFAVb

Essential Oils Box Set #9 Essential Oil and Weight Loss & Carrier Oils

http://amzn.to/1jmcEPP

Essential Oils Box Set #10 Hyperthyroidism Manual & Hypothyroidism Manual

http://amzn.to/1nHgJU4

Essential Oils Box Set #11 Carrier Oils for Beginners & Coconut Oil for Easy Weight Loss

http://amzn.to/1nHfy6X

Essential Oils Box Set #12 Essential Oils Weight Loss & Essential Oils Aromatherapy & Natural Homemade Cleaning Supplies & Top Essential Oil Recipes & Carrier Oils
http://amzn.to/1nHfy6X

Essential Oils Box Set #13 Superfoods & Essential Weight Loss & Essential Aromatherapy & Body Butters & Soap Making
http://amzn.to/1nUds6v

Essential Oils Box Set #14 Weight Loss & Apple Cider Vinegar & Body Butters & Homemade Body Scrubs & Coconut Oil for Beginners
http://amzn.to/1i1qYOd

Essential Oils Box Set #15 The Beginners Guide To Making your Own Essential Oils & The Beginners Guide to Medicinal Plants
http://amzn.to/1m6wNC4

Essential Oils Box Set #16 Thyroid Diet & Hypothyroidism Handbook
http://amzn.to/1wmtIOI

Essential Oils Box Set #17 Top Essential Oil Recipes & The Beginners Guide to Making Your Own Essential Oils
http://amzn.to/1BGYhBu

If the links do not work, for whatever reason, you can simply search for these titles on the Amazon website to find them.

www.ingramcontent.com/pod-product-compliance
Lightning Source LLC
Chambersburg PA
CBHW070459290526
45790CB00003B/1020